Welcome to the
"Conversations About Nurse Bullying" Toolkit

The purpose of this Toolkit is to provide schools of nursing and healthcare organizations with the resources and strategies to:

1. Prepare pre-licensure nursing students and newly licensed nurses for the reality of disruptive behavior in the current healthcare environment,
2. Set expectations for professional behavior to help prevent the next generation of nurse bullies, and
3. Provide practical strategies to address disruptive behavior in the work environment.

Each chapter includes objectives, an optional group activity and a list of questions that can be used in a live or online forum. Feel free to use these exercises as written or modify to meet the course objectives.

How to use this Toolkit:
- Ensure that each student/newly licensed nurse receives a copy of the book, "Do No Harm" Applies to Nurses Too! Strategies to protect and bully-proof yourself at work **(see bulk book order form on page 37)**.
- Review the objectives, activities, and discussion questions for each chapter. Select questions and activities that best fit the needs of your organization. Depending on your academic/residency calendar, these questions can be used in the classroom setting, post-conference sessions during clinical rotations, throughout orientation and within an online discussion format.
- Allow the students/newly licensed nurses time (at least once a week) to read each chapter before participating in the coordinating discussion questions.

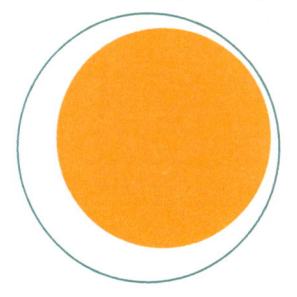

This Toolkit is copyright by RTConnections and cannot be shared beyond the licensing agreement parameters.

© 2014 RTConnections, LLC   rtconnections.com

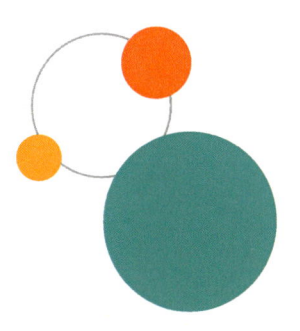

TABLE OF CONTENTS

	PAGE
CHAPTER 1: NURSES ARE EATING THEIR YOUNG - EVERYWHERE	5
CHAPTER 2: MEET THE BULLY FAMILY	9
CHAPTER 3: BULLYING ATTRACTIVE FACTORS - WHO MAKES A GOOD TARGET?	13
CHAPTER 4: LAYING THE FOUNDATION TO PROTECT YOURSELF	17
CHAPTER 5: THE "WHY" BEHIND NURSE BULLY BEHAVIOR	21
CHAPTER 6: PROFILES OF THE BULLY NURSES YOU MAY KNOW	25
CHAPTER 7: STEPS TO STOP THE BULLYING	27
CHAPTER 8: WHEN ENOUGH IS ENOUGH	31
CHAPTER 9: WHAT TO DO IF THE BULLY IS YOU	35
CHAPTER 10: IT'S TIME FOR EVERYONE TO ACT	37
ATTACHMENT A	39
ATTACHMENT B	41
ATTACHMENT C	47
ATTACHMENT D	49
RESOURCES	53
BULK ORDER FORM	55

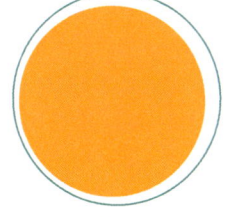

CHAPTER 1: NURSES ARE EATING THEIR YOUNG - EVERYWHERE

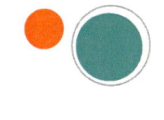

Objectives:

By the end of this chapter, students/newly licensed nurses will be able to:

1. Examine personal attitudes and responses towards bullying in the workplace
2. Relate the acts of bullying to an unhealthy work environment.
3. Identify issues related to the development of institutional and national policies to address bullying behavior in the healthcare setting
4. Contrast acts of bullying to the provisions in the ANA Code of Ethics for Nurses.

Group Activity: Option 1

Materials: None

Timeframe: 20-30 minutes

Instructions: Divide class into groups of 3-5. Ask each student/newly-licensed nurse to share a story where they've either experienced or witnessed bullying behavior by a nurse. Ask each group to select one story to share with the class.

Group Activity: Option 2

Materials: ANA Code of Ethics for Nurses

Time Frame: 30 minutes

Instructions: Have students review the ANA Code of Ethics for Nurses. Relate the provisions to bullying behaviors they may have seen or engaged in. Use the following questions for discussion:

1. Which of the following provisions are violated when bullying occurs in nursing?
2. How does this impact the profession as a whole?
3. Could nurse bullying alter the way other professions see nursing?
4. What impact might this have on the manner other professions treat nurses?

Discussion Questions:

1. The author describes "Cathy", a nurse bully. Have you experienced anyone like Cathy during your clinical rotations? If so, please describe your experience.

2. Refer to page 3 of the book. The author provides examples of bullying behavior. Share a situation when you've experienced or witnessed similar behaviors in the clinical environment. How did it make you feel? How did you respond? Did anyone respond? If so, how?

3. There is a quote from President Barack Obama on page 5: "We've got to dispel the myth that bullying is a rite of passage." Do you believe that in nursing, it is an expectation for new nurses to suffer some level of bullying? Is bullying in nursing considered "normal" or a rite of passage? How does this impact the learning environment

4. "Zero Tolerance" policies are being instituted at many facilities. Do you think nursing schools should also have this policy? Is there a need for a policy that directly addresses bullying? If so, what kinds of things should be included as part of that policy?

5. Discuss "Kaitlin's" story on pages 8-9. What is your first impression of Kaitlin? What is your impression of the nurses on the unit? What would you do if you were in Kaitlin's situation?

6. The author describes the impact bullying has on individuals, organizations, the nursing profession, and patients. Share your thoughts on that impact and provide examples that support her claims.

7. Did anyone warn you about "nurses eating their young"? If so, who? Did you consider changing your career because of the concerns about this? Do you know anyone who perhaps wanted to become a nurse, but didn't want to work in a "hostile" environment?

8. The author suggests that to begin the journey to a "world where bullying doesn't exist" is to begin with developing moral courage. Describe what moral courage means to you. Have you ever been in a situation when you've had to do something, were afraid but did it anyway? Can you relate this experience to moral courage?

9. The author suggests a "world where bullying doesn't exist. Where nurses go out of their way to support each other...." Do you believe this world is possible?

CHAPTER 2: MEET THE BULLY FAMILY

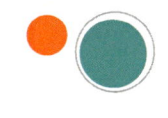

Objectives:

By the end of this chapter, students/newly licensed nurses will be able to:

1. Identify the three terms used to describe bullying
2. Compare and contrast overt and covert behaviors
3. Give examples of behaviors that may be considered bullying

Group Activity: Overt and Covert Bullying

Timeframe: 30 minutes

Materials: Index cards with a list of behaviors (see Attachment A)

Divide the class into groups of 3-5. Place the index cards face down in a pile. Ask each student/newly-licensed nurse to choose a card, read the behavior out loud, and identify if the behavior is considered overt or covert. Encourage the students/newly-licensed nurses to dialogue, sharing their experiences with that behavior.

Discussion Questions:

1. Complete the assessment on page 17, "Assess your Experience with Bullying." Were you surprised with your results? What behaviors did you experience that you didn't realize could be considered bullying?
2. When did you first hear the term horizontal violence used in the nursing profession? Describe your reaction.
3. Did you ever question your ability to become a successful nurse because of horizontal violence?
4. Explain the difference between overt and covert behaviors and provide examples of each from your experience.
5. On page 20, the author includes a table of overt and covert bullying behaviors. Which of these

behaviors have you experienced more often? Please share an example.

6. In your opinion, is one (overt or covert) more harmful than the other? Please explain.

7. Read the story about Lisa on pages 21-23. How do you think you would have handled Norma if you were in the same situation? What could Lisa have done to protect herself from Norma?

8. Read the story about Susan on pages 24-25. What bullying behavior did Susan's colleagues use? (Answer: Exclusion) What could Susan have done to address their behaviors? What would you do if you found yourself in a similar situation?

9. Why do you think some nurses downplay other nurses' accomplishments? Have you seen this in your environment?

10. Complete the "Action Step" on page 28 and share your results with your colleagues.

CHAPTER 3: BULLYING ATTRACTIVE FACTORS - WHO MAKES A GOOD TARGET?

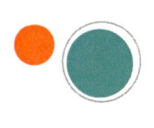

Objectives:

By the end of this chapter, students/newly licensed nurses will be able to:

1. Relate common behaviors in the workplace that increase a person's chance of becoming a target of bullying
2. Describe the four communication styles and provide an example of each
3. Generate three strategies or behaviors that can decrease a person's chance of becoming a target of bullying

Group Activity: Communication Style Role-Playing (see Attachment B)

Materials: Handouts (Attachment B)

Timeframe: 30 minutes

Divide the class into groups of 5-6. Provide each group with a scenario and ask the groups to role-play a response using the different communication styles.

Discussion Questions:

1. In Chapter 3, the author starts by telling the reader to STOP! She suggests that many victims of bullying blame themselves. Have you personally experienced self-blame before? Can you describe your feelings as they relate to self-blame?
2. The author relates the targets of bullying to the victims of crimes. Share your thoughts on this comparison. Do you see similarities? Are there major differences?
3. Displaying diminished self-confidence is a behavior that the author suggests attracts a bully. What characteristics and behaviors do you believe exist in someone who suffers from diminished self-confidence? What behaviors have you seen in someone who appears confident?

4. Read the story about Diane on pages 35-36. Has a "Carol" ever treated you in a similar manner? If so, how did you handle it? What role did the physician play in Diane's ability to ward off attacks from future "Carols"? What types of actions could you employ that would help avoid becoming/remaining a victim?

5. According to the author, displaying passive behavior and communication style is a "bully attractive factor". Describe examples of passive behavior and communication you've witnessed in your personal and professional environments.

6. The author shares the four different communication styles. Which one do you see most often in the healthcare environment? Share examples of each with your peers.

7. Answer questions on page 40 - evaluating communication styles. Discuss the various options, including the type of communication style and the pros/cons of using this style. Is there power in how we respond to situations?

8. Walking a different path is identified as putting a nurse at risk for bullying. What differences have you witnessed in your environment that might put someone at risk for bullying?

9. The author suggests that being different can put you at risk for bullying, even if you communicate using the assertive style. Read the story about Laura on pages 45-46. Share your thoughts on Laura's situation. Consider if Laura used the passive communication style, how might her story have changed?

10. On page 49, the author includes a list of behaviors that help to decrease your chances of becoming a target of bullying. Which three behaviors do you believe have the most impact on combating bullying? Are there any behaviors you could add? How can we minimize these factors and decrease the targets for bullies?

CHAPTER 4: LAYING THE FOUNDATION TO PROTECT YOURSELF

Objectives:

By the end of this chapter, students/newly licensed nurses will be able to:

1. Discuss three strategies to decrease a person's chance of becoming a target of bullying
2. Evaluate characteristics of assertive communication
3. Formulate a plan that will allow a person to respond appropriately to comments regarding differences

Group Activity: Bully-Proofing Strategies (See Attachment C)

Materials: Handouts

Timeframe: 20 minutes

Provide each student/newly-licensed nurse with a copy of Attachment C. Give the students 10 minutes to complete the exercise. Ask for volunteers who will share their results. Engage students/newly licensed nurses in dialogue regarding bully-proofing strategies.

Discussion Questions:

1. Describe a time when you felt insecure about a task or activity you needed to do. What characteristics did you display?
2. Eye contact is an important strategy to appear to be more self-confident. Are you comfortable looking others in the eye when interacting with them? Why do you think some people avoid eye contact? What is your impression of someone who doesn't look you in the eye?
3. Dressing professionally is described as a bully-proofing strategy. Why do you think this is an important strategy to decrease your chances of becoming a target? Do you agree or disagree with the author? Please support your response
4. Think about voicing your opinion as a new nurse. Are you comfortable speaking-up for yourself

if you are in an uncomfortable situation? How can you respectfully voice your opinion without appearing confrontational? What situations could you find yourself in where you may need to speak-up for yourself?

5. On pages 56 – 61, the author provides examples of assertive and non-assertive communication. Review the examples and discuss. Share examples you've seen in your environment of assertive communication. Share examples you've seen in your environment of non-assertive communication.

6. Read the story about Valerie on pages 61-62. Were you surprised to learn that bullying occurs in other positions beyond the bedside? What bully-proofing strategy did Valerie use to stop being "dumped" on by the other educators? Is this something you could do in a similar situation?

7. The author suggests engaging in positive self-talk as a strategy to become more assertive. Provide a few examples of positive self-talk statements you could rehearse as a student/newly licensed nurse or new nurse.

8. Read the story about Jan on pages 63-65. Have you ever been in a situation where someone openly criticized you in front of others for something not completely within your responsibility? How did you feel while being openly criticized? What bully-proofing strategy did Jan use to address the CNO? Is this a strategy you believe you could use if in a similar situation? If not, why not?

9. Identify one difference you have that may set you apart from your nursing colleagues. How would you respond if someone treated you poorly because of this difference?

10. Discuss gender differences. Do you still see male and female nurses being treated differently? How? If so, why do you think this happens? What could you do to encourage acceptance of both male and female nurses?

CHAPTER 5: THE "WHY" BEHIND NURSE BULLY BEHAVIOR

Objectives:

By the end of this chapter, students/newly licensed nurses will be able to:

1. Describe three theories regarding why nurse bullying occurs
2. Correlate underlying personal characteristics with bullying behavior
3. Characterize behaviors commonly seen in passive-aggressive communication styles

Discussion Questions:

1. The author describes the nursing profession as an oppressed group. Do you agree or disagree? Please support your response.

2. Do you believe nurses are still treated as servants lacking any real decision-making or power in their role? Can you share an example of when you've witnessed nurses treated in this way?

3. Read Sarah's story on pages 72-73. Why do you think Sarah gave up trying to improve things and became a bully? What else could Sarah have done? Does learning about the reason Sarah became a bully help you feel compassion for her?

4. Female-to-female aggression is described. What examples have you seen in your environment, personally or professionally, where females engage in unhealthy competition? Alternatively, share examples of healthy competition among females.

5. Low self-esteem has been identified as a primary reason why nurses bully. However, the author suggests that some bullies actually have high self-esteem; and therefore, bully others because they think they are superior. What are your thoughts on this premise?

6. The author suggests that bullies, who are of the Millennial Generation, are more likely to have issues with high self-esteem. Do you agree or disagree?

7. What role do generational differences play in the way nurses treat each other?

8. Read the quote by Tom Hiddleston on page 77. If the bully started as a victim, does it change how you perceive him or her?

9. The author describes the characteristics of aggressive behavior. Share an example of aggressive behavior you've witnessed in the clinical setting. Describe the body language and any behaviors that can be labeled as aggressive.

10. The author describes the characteristics of passive-aggressive behavior. Have you ever communicated using this style? Think about why you choose to communicate in this way. Can you identify the reasons? What would have been a better communication style to use in that situation?

CHAPTER 6: PROFILES OF THE BULLY NURSES YOU MAY KNOW

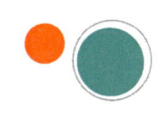

Objectives:

By the end of this chapter, students/newly licensed nurses will be able to:

1. Describe which profile types utilize overt or covert behavior as their primary method
2. Differentiate various characteristics of each bullying profile

Group Activity:

Materials: None

Timeframe: 30 minutes

In this chapter, the primary activity is to engage the students/newly-licensed nurses in open discussion regarding bully profiles. For each profile type, ask the students/newly-licensed nurses to share examples and to engage in dialogue about the unique behaviors. This should be done as a class activity.

Super Nurse _____

Energy Vampire _____

Viper Nurse _____

Sorority Nurse _____

Bitter Nurse _____

CHAPTER 7: STEPS TO STOP THE BULLYING

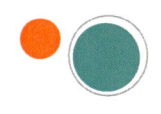

Objectives:

By the end of this chapter, students/newly licensed nurses will be able to:

1. Summarize the four steps to stop bullying
2. Construct a plan with at least three interventions to address overt bullying behavior
3. Construct a plan with at least three interventions to address covert bullying behavior

Group Activity: Role Playing

Practice Confronting the Bully: Assign each group a scenario throughout the book (Cathy page 1; Kaitlin page 8; Norma, page 22; Susan, page 24; Eric, page 48. Using the four steps to stop bullying, ask each group to develop a plan for their scenario.

Discussion Questions:

Discuss the various steps to stop bullying:

1. Recognize you are a victim: Describe the environment when a bully is present. Are other people also victims? Do you think some people may have difficulty with this step? Why? (Reflect on "June and Frank".) Looking back on your interactions with others, can you now identify situations as bullying that you didn't realize were bullying before?

    a. Separate yourself mentally from the bully: Think again about the environment during a bullying exchange. Describe the anxiety level you may have felt during such an exchange. Perhaps you have observed another person being bullied.

    b. Describe the environment. How do we detach ourselves from the bully's behavior?

    c. Speak up: Can you identify a mentor that you can go to if you experience bullying? The book lists possibilities as preceptors, nurse educators, colleagues, or a friend. Can you identify any others? What are the risks of speaking up? What are the benefits?

d. Confront the bully: How difficult is it to "name the behavior" when the bully is in a position of authority? What can you do in this case?

2. What does moral courage mean to you? What role does moral courage play in the ability to stop bullying behavior? What steps can you take to strengthen moral courage?

3. Read the quote by Eleanor Roosevelt on page 96. What does this quote mean to you? Share an example of when you allowed someone else to make you feel bad about yourself.

4. Read the story about Courtney on pages 102-103. What were the steps Courtney used to end the bullying? Do you believe these steps would work for you? What barriers exist?

5. The author provides examples of "naming the behavior" as a strategy to confront the bully. Can you think of other examples you could use? Notice that naming the behavior can be used for both overt and covert behaviors. How are they similar? How are they different?

6. Walking away from an overt bully is a strategy to address bullying behavior. Have you ever walked away from someone who was yelling or openly criticizing you? Do you think walking away requires moral courage? How likely is it that you could implement this strategy if faced with an overt bully?

7. The author indicates that although confronting doesn't always work, failure to confront NEVER works. What impact does failure to confront have on the nursing profession? Is it sometimes better to avoid and not confront a bully?

CHAPTER 8: WHEN ENOUGH IS ENOUGH

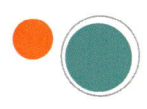

Objectives:

By the end of this chapter, students/newly licensed nurses will be able to:

1. Examine various strategies a witness can implement to stop bullying behavior and discuss potential outcomes

2. Summarize the role of the manager in eliminating bullying

3. Compare and contrast the working environment in which bullying occurs with that of a healthy work environment

Group Activity: How would you respond? (See Attachment D)

Discussion Questions:

1. The author suggests that there is a difference between complaining and filing a complaint. Discuss the difference and share any examples from your experience.

2. The author recommends that if you've done your part (recognize, separate, speak up and confront) and the bullying behavior continues, leaving the unit and/or organization is necessary. Do you believe this is a valid step? What repercussions would result? What would stop you from leaving despite being bullied?

3. Page 115 includes a statistic about witnessing bullying behavior. Do these numbers surprise you? Have you ever seen a nurse intervene when someone is being bullied? Do you think you could intervene if you witness a bully attack?

4. The author talks about establishing goals that encompass the ideal work environment. Two aspects of this environment include: demonstrating respect and support. Identify ways, in this clinical group and in the classroom, where respect was demonstrated. Also, where support was demonstrated.

5. Have you seen/taken part in a lack of respect for others? A lack of support? How did this affect the clinical group or class as a whole?

6. The author includes recommendations for managers to eliminate bullying behavior. In your opinion, what role does the manager play in promoting or eliminating bullying? Should managers set expectations for behavior in addition to performance?

7. What role does the manager have in holding employees accountable? What role do the employees have in holding each other accountable?

8. Discuss peer-to-peer accountability and how this might impact the work environment. How comfortable or uncomfortable would you be in addressing the bad behavior or performance of your peer? Has anyone addressed YOUR bad behavior or performance? How did it make you feel? How did you react?

CHAPTER 9: WHAT TO DO IF THE BULLY IS YOU

Objectives:

By the end of this chapter, students/newly licensed nurses will be able to:

1. Give three examples of bullying behaviors
2. Develop two strategies that can be incorporated into practice that will allow an individual to leave a herd

Group Activity:

Materials: None

Timeframe: 30 minutes

Watch the slide show located on the Stanford Prison Experiment website: http://www.prisonexp.org. Ask the students/newly licensed nurses to share their insights with their peers. What did they find most shocking? How do they think they would react if found in a similar situation?

Discussion Questions:

1. Complete "Bully Behavior Assessment" found on page 129. Were you surprised by the findings? How often are these behaviors the result of the environment (Carly example)?
2. What can you do now that you have identified these behaviors? How can the environment be changed to one of support and not bullying?
3. Have you ever considered that you might be contributing to nurse bullying?
4. Have you ever behaved in a way that was different than your personality to fit in with others? Reflect on your experience. What would have happened if you didn't go along with the crowd/herd?
5. Read the section on dropping out of the herd on pages 133-136. If you found yourself as part of a bullying herd, what strategy could you adopt to drop out of the herd? Which strategy do you believe will be the most difficult?

CHAPTER 10: IT'S TIME FOR EVERYONE TO ACT

Objectives:

By the end of this chapter, students/newly licensed nurses will be able to:

1. Outline three action steps to take if you are the target of bullying
2. Outline three action steps to take if you are the witness of bullying
3. Construct a strategy you can implement if you realize you engage in bullying behavior

Activity:

Ask each participant to create an individualized action plan based on the content in Chapter 10.

Discussion Questions:

1. On page 138, the author categorizes people into one of three categories. Which category do you fit in? Are there other categories you would include?
2. Which action steps do you believe would be most successful if you found yourself as the target of bullying?
3. Regarding "reporting to an authority figure", how likely is it that you would report bullying behavior? What would be the risk involved?
4. Discuss the issue of retaliation. Have you experienced retaliation from someone? What steps could you take to minimize the impact of retaliation?
5. Do you believe you are now better prepared to address bullying behavior in the work environment?
6. What are your key take-aways from this book? How will you use them in your current environment? How will you use them when you start your first job as a nurse?

ATTACHMENT A

Chapter 2: Group Activity: Overt and Covert Behavior

Objective: Help student/graduate nurses recognize the differences between overt and covert behavior.

Materials: Behavior index cards. Words can be written on index cards or printed on labels and attached. Include the word(s) only. Do not identify behavior as overt or covert on the cards.

Timeframe: 30 minutes

Facilitator instructions: Divide participants into groups of 3-5. Allow groups to sit together in a circle. Place the index cards faced down. Each member in the group draws from the index card pile. Each card has a word(s) that can be considered overt or covert behavior. The participants should read their word(s) aloud, identify if it's an overt or covert behavior and then share an experience.

Words:

Overt	Covert
Yelling	Excluding others
Criticizing	Withholding information
Bickering	Assigning unfair workloads
Blaming	Refusing to help
Raising eyebrows	Taking credit for somebody else's work
Rolling eyes	Undermining
Gossiping	Using sarcasm
Threatening others	Downplaying accomplishments

All additional behaviors based on your current environment

Instructor tips:

The key learning objective is to help the students/newly licensed nurses identify behaviors and to categorize them as either overt or covert. Please note: There are some behaviors, such as eye rolling, which can be categorized as overt or covert depending on the situation (see page 27). Encourage the students/graduate nurses to identify other behaviors they have witnessed that are not on the list.

ATTACHMENT B

Chapter 3: Group Activity

Communication Styles

Objective: To identify characteristics of the four communication styles in common scenarios.

Materials: Scenarios

Timeframe: 30 minutes

Facilitator instructions: Divide participants into groups of 5-6. Give each group a scenario. Each group is to develop a response based on each communication style (passive, aggressive, passive-aggressive, assertive).

Scenario #1

Assignments are due by the end of the day. A classmate (and friend) approaches you asking for help to complete hers. You are also having a very busy day, and are on a tight timeline. How will you respond using the four different communication styles?

Passive:

Aggressive:

Passive-Aggressive:

Assertive:

Scenario #2

Your clinical instructor asks you to create a bulletin board highlighting the newest CPR guidelines. You create a dynamic bulletin board. You overhear your instructor taking full credit for the "great job". How will you respond using the four different communication styles?

Passive:

Aggressive:

Passive-Aggressive:

Assertive:

Scenario #3

A terrible storm blasts through your city prompting the school to close. You are thankful that you don't have to go to class in the storm; however, this class was the last class prior to the exam. Although your instructor provides a study guide for the exam, you and many of your classmates do poorly. Your classmates blame the instructor for not providing sufficient guidance on the study guide and are planning to complain to the dean. You believe the instructor should not be blamed for the poor grades.

Using the four communication styles, how do you respond?

Passive:

Aggressive:

Passive-Aggressive:

Assertive:

Scenario #4

You are assignment a patient on the clinical unit. When you approach Tina the nurse and tell her you're a student assigned to her patient, she rolls her eyes and says loudly, "Why do I have to get a student?"

Using the four communication styles, how do you respond?

Passive:

Aggressive:

Passive-Aggressive:

Assertive:

Scenario #5

You think you have a good relationship with the other students in your clinical rotation. However, one of your peers tells you that whenever you walk out of the room, two of your classmates start making fun of you and criticizing you.

Using the four communication styles, how do you respond?

Passive:

Aggressive:

Passive-Aggressive:

Assertive:

ATTACHMENT C

Chapter 4: Activity

Bully-proofing actions

Objective: Create an action plan of behaviors to decrease chances of becoming a bully's target.

Materials: Handout

Timeframe: 10-15 minutes

Chapter 4 discusses bully-proofing yourself and lists several techniques. Which of the following do you currently use? Which could you adopt?

#1 Project Self Confidence	Currently Use	Could Adopt
Look people in the eye		
Walk tall, sit tall		
Dress professionally		
- Follow dress code		
- Wear patient appropriate attire		
- Neat, clean, pressed		
Voice your opinion		
Act as if…		

Select one of these methods above that you will incorporate. Share with your peers.

#2 Practice Assertive Behavior / Communucation	Currently Use	Could Adopt
Use cooperative words		
Display an even, confident voice		
Give specific descriptions		
Use open / honest statements		
Actively listen		
Focus on the issue, not the person		
Use non-judgmental communication		
Actively communicates expectations		

Select one of these methods above that you will incorporate. Share with your peers.

© 2014 RTConnections, LLC   rtconnections.com

ATTACHMENT D

Chapter 8: Group Activity

How do you respond?

Objective: To prepare responses to common situations involving disruptive behavior.

Materials: Scenarios

Timeframe: 30 minutes

Facilitator instructions: Share the following situations with your students/nurses. Ask how they might respond to each situation.

Situations:

1. You overhear a nurse call your colleague an idiot in front of everyone at the nurses' station.

    HOW DO YOU RESPOND?

2. Several co-workers are bullying you. Although you've complained to your manager, to your knowledge, nothing has been done.

    HOW DO YOU RESPOND?

3. Your colleague confides in you that he is being bullied by several of the older, female nurses. According to your colleague, these nurses make sexual remarks towards him, share inappropriate jokes, and give him the worst assignments when in charge.

    HOW DO YOU RESPOND?

© 2014 RTConnections, LLC

4. A physician demands to see "the nurse caring for Mr. Rossi." When you are asked to speak with him, he starts screaming at you because the lab work he ordered wasn't done.

   HOW DO YOU RESPOND?

5. You find out that one of your colleagues has been saying negative things about you when you're not there.

   HOW DO YOU RESPOND?

PRODUCTS

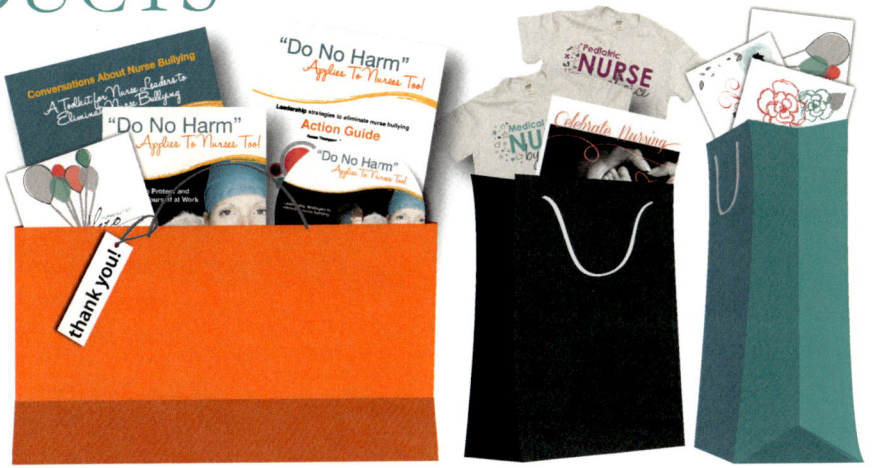

ADDITIONAL RESOURCES

To purchase Renee's products, go to: rtconnections.com/products

KEYNOTES & SEMINARS

SEMINARS

"Do No Harm" Applies to Nurses Too!
Strategies to protect and
bully-proof yourself at work

**Communication, Conflict
and Co-workers – Oh My!**
Navigating the Yellow-brick Road
to Effective Communication

**Navigating the Social Media
Super Highway**
Strategies for nurse leaders

KEYNOTES

Celebrate Nursing:
Human by birth – Hero by choice

From Exhausted to Extraordinary!
Strategies to Reverse Nurse Fatigue

Navigating the Road to Exemplary Practice

Harnessing the Power of Social Media:
Strategies for Nurse Leaders

"Do No Harm" Applies to Nurses Too!
Strategies to protect and bully-proof yourself at work

BRING ANY OF RENEE'S SEMINARS OR PRESENTATIONS TO **YOUR** ORGANIZATION!

CERTIFICATION COURSES:

- Medical Surgical Certification Review Course
- Critical Care Certification Review Course
- Certified Emergency Nurse Review Course
- CPAN/CAPA Certification Review Course

412.445.2653 | renee@rtconnections.com

rtconnections.com

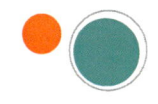

Since you purchased Renee's **"Conversations About Nurse Bullying"** Toolkit, you are entitled to DISCOUNT PRICES....
on the book **"Do No Harm" Applies To Nurses Too!**

Order yours today!
Save by buying "Do No Harm" Applies to Nurses Too! in bulk. *(Retail Price $19.97)*

Quantity	Discounted Price
1 – 25	$18 / book
26 – 50	$16 / book
51 – 100	$14 / book
>100	$12 / book

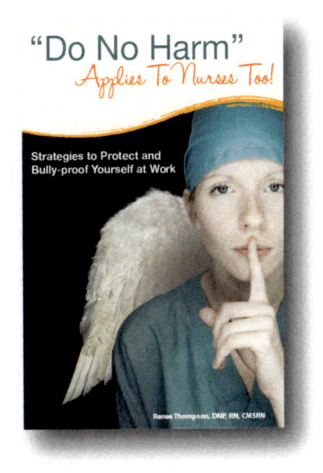

BEST DEAL!

ORDERING OPTIONS:
- complete form and mail to RTConnections: 146, Aidan Ct, Pittsburgh PA 15226
- complete and scan to RTConnections via email renee@rtconnections.com
- call Renee at 412.445.2653

To invite Renee to your organization to present, **"Do No Harm" Applies To Nurses Too!** please contact her at: renee@rtconnections.com or call 412.445.2653

ORDER FORM

Name: DAWNA RUTHERFORD
Address: 3405 MIDDLETON AVE #79
City: CINCINNATI   State: OH   Zip: 45220
Phone: 757-274-9018   Email: RUTHERDA@mail.uc.edu or (DAWNA6970@AOL.COM)

Number of books ordered: 10

PAYMENT OPTIONS:
☒ CREDIT CARD ☐ CHECK   Make check payable to: RTConnections, LLC
(Mail to: 146 Aidan Court, Pittsburgh PA 15226)

Name on card: DAWNA RUTHERFORD
Card number: 4092 6372 9015 8658   Expiration date: 09 / 2020
3 digit security code: 770   Billing Zip: 45220

© 2014 RTConnections, LLC   rtconnections.com

Made in the USA
Middletown, DE
19 June 2018